Breastfeeding
an Adopted Baby and Relactation

LA LECHE LEAGUE INTERNATIONAL

written and translated by
Elizabeth Hormann, IBCLC

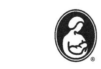

LA LECHE LEAGUE
INTERNATIONAL

Schaumburg, IL

First printing, November 2006
  German Edition © 1989, 1998, E. Hormann
  English Edition © 2005, 2006, Eliz Hormann
All rights reserved
Printed in the United States of America
Book and cover design Patricia Gager

Photo credits
Allen Morgan, cover photo
John Osytn 6, 42
Márta Guóth-Gumberger 10, 21, 24, 26, 27, 32,
36, 38, 46, 50
Mimi de Maza 37
Molly Davis 12
Pamela Willett 16, 44
Susan Cooper 52

Author and translator: Elizabeth Hormann, IBCLC

ISBN-10: 0-9768969-7-4
ISBN-13: 978-0-9768969-7-5
Library of Congress Card Number 2005937925

La Leche League International
P.O. Box 4079
Schaumburg, IL 60168-4079
www.llli.org

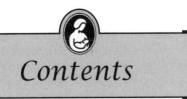

Contents

Dedication

This book is dedicated to Robert and Willi, my first foster sons, and most especially to Charles Alexander Yorck Hormann, my son by adoption. I have learned from all three of you—now grown men—and with you, I have experienced breastfeeding as a real gift.

Special thanks to

Renate Pasch—who helped me with the first translation into German in 1989;

Barbara Herrmann—who did the German language corrections;

Denise Both, Frauke Bratz, Cordelia Koppitz, Maria Rost, and Eva Stroh—who read through the German manuscript and put it into its final form;

Márta Guóth-Gumberger and Rudi Gumberger—who read and commented on the manuscript for both the German and the English editions;

Cordelia Koppitz, Denise Both, and Diana West—who reviewed the English manuscript; and

Nancy Jo Bykowski—LLLI language editor.

Foreword

As I held my first adopted baby in my arms, I was given Elizabeth Hormann's telephone number by La Leche League. The conversations with her became a precious part of my life.

She advised me and was at my side, sensitively, professionally, through many long telephone calls, from the first tentative breastfeeding attempts through the long years of breastfeeding three adopted children, exploring with me not only breastfeeding, but also the basic issues of adoption and childrearing.

She left her mark not only on me as a mother, but also on my own breastfeeding counseling later on. With her I experienced continual loving respect for children, fathers, and above all for mothers. This respect embraced both the adoptive mother and the mother who had given birth to the child. Out of this grew a way of counseling that looked at the actual conditions realistically and, at the same time, supported the mother in her role without any pressure to achieve a specific result.

You will find this viewpoint between the lines of the book that you hold in your hands. This makes the comprehensive and relevant information about adoptive breastfeeding particularly valuable. This book provides not only evidence-based professional information, but also decision-making help, motivation, and encouragement for the mother and those who are supporting her, whatever decisions are made.

The German language edition of this book was one of the first comprehensive publications on this topic. While other publications have appeared in English since the author issued the very first breastfeeding guide for adoptive mothers in 1971, this book remains unique because of its combination of professional and practical information presented in a warm, informal style.

I hope this book will be useful for many adoptive mothers as well as breastfeeding counselors and others interested in supporting these mothers, and that it will enable many adoptive mothers and their babies to enjoy the experience of breastfeeding.

Márta Guóth-Gumberger

Introduction

When the subject of breastfeeding an adopted baby comes up, eyebrows often go up as well. Even though the trend in the latter part of the twentieth century and into this one has been to encourage breastfeeding, that encouragement has rarely extended to the adoptive mother and her baby. Breastfeeding is seen—and rightly so—as a natural extension of the pregnancy and birth process. But to see it **only** in this light is to take too narrow a view both of the concept of breastfeeding and of the biological possibilities.

Breastfeeding a baby is more than just feeding. It provides a close intimate interaction between mother and baby that involves all the senses. Mother and baby are in touch, skin-to-skin. They may spend part of the breastfeeding time gazing into each other's eyes. Mothers talk and croon to their babies while they breastfeed, and babies, from a very early age, make little noises that even the most inexperienced mother recognizes as sounds of satisfaction. Breastfed babies are drawn to their mothers' breasts in part by smell (within a few days after birth they can distinguish their mothers from other women by smell alone). And babies, like other people, also enjoy their food because of its taste.

Mothers enjoy that sweet baby smell (all the sweeter if he is being breastfed) and what mother has not indulged in a little finger nibbling as she has held her baby close? These interactions are not exclusive to breastfeeding couples. Many bottle-feeding mothers and their babies enjoy very close contact with one another, but this contact is built into the breastfeeding relationship in an easy comfortable way that is quickly picked up even when both mother and baby are amateurs.

Adoptive mothers, like mothers of homegrown children, may also want to have the sort of relationship with their babies that breastfeeding offers. For the mother adopting because she has been unable to conceive or carry a baby to term, breastfeeding may offer a share in the biological experiences of motherhood that have otherwise passed her by.

There are special benefits for the baby as well. His entrance into the world, no matter how carefully and lovingly arranged by his birth parents and his adoptive parents, has not been easy. He has been separated from the mother whose heartbeat and voice and body rhythms he knew and he has had to make an attachment to a new mother who is, at first, a complete stranger. This attachment is far easier to make if he spends a good deal of his time in her arms, skin-to-skin, close to her heart. There he grows familiar with and learns to love the sounds of her heart and her voice, the feel of her skin on his, her special sweet smell and the face that he will soon prefer above all others.

Breastfeeding has some physical advantages for the adopted baby as well, though they may not be as extensive as they are for a baby who has been born to his mother. Even a small amount of milk (and nearly all adoptive mothers will have some) can be helpful in protecting against allergies and provides nutrition that is ideally suited not just to babies in general, but to this baby in particular. The baby's mouth at the breast sends subtle signals that ensure that his mother's milk is suited to his developmental stage and has antibodies to the illnesses to which both mother and baby have been exposed.

The baby who suckles at the breast regularly—even if his primary nourishment comes from another source—is using his jaw and facial muscles the way they were meant to be used. He learns to position his tongue correctly at the gum line and to swallow in the way a baby should. The habits he learns suckling at the breast can have a profound effect on the positioning of his permanent teeth and on the development of his speech. Alternating from one breast to another is important for the development of hand-eye coordination. Convenience is not usually so much of an advantage in breastfeeding an adoptive baby as it is in breastfeeding a child you have borne yourself, but if the baby breastfeeds for comfort or to go to sleep, it is just as convenient for adoptive families at these times as it is for any other family.

Breastfeeding an adopted baby or relactating for a homegrown baby is not easy. It requires time, strong commitment, a good bit of patience, and as much support as you can muster. This option may not suit every family or every baby adopted into a family. But for many families, there are some compelling advantages. This book provides accurate information and strong support to get you started and to keep you going.

Definitions:

Induced lactation vs. relactation

From a medical perspective, the adoptive mother who breastfeeds her baby may induce lactation (i.e., lactate without a prior pregnancy and birth) or she may relactate (i.e., re-establish lactation after a gap of several weeks, months, or years). Strictly speaking, it is the woman who has never been pregnant who induces lactation. A woman who has had a baby—no matter how long ago it was—relactates when she brings in a milk supply for an adopted baby or for a homegrown baby who didn't get started at breastfeeding right after birth (Hormann and Savage 1998; Lawrence 2005).

For our purposes here, we will consider that a woman is inducing lactation—even if she has previously given birth—provided that she is not lactating at all when she begins breastfeeding or bringing in a milk supply, and it has been at least six months since she last lactated. If you weaned, had a miscarriage, an abortion, a stillbirth, lost a newborn baby, or didn't breastfeed at all after your last birth and it has been more than six months since one of these events took place, the information about induced lactation is meant for you. If it has been less than six months, the sections on relactation will probably be most relevant to your situation.

In Chapters 2 through 7 and in Chapters 9 and 10, you will find information that is particularly helpful for relactation.

Chapter 1
Myths about Breastfeeding an Adopted Baby:
A Historical Overview

Breastfeeding your adopted baby—or even talking about the possibility —may cause a stir in your family, among your neighbors, at the adoption agency, and in your doctor's office. Myths about it generally fall into three categories:

No one does it.

It is inappropriate.

It is impossible.

Myth 1: No one does it

While breastfeeding is by no means a routine part of adoption, neither is it a rarity. My first study in 1971 included 27 women. The second studied 65 different women (out of 75 respondents to a questionnaire). Over more than 30 years, I have collected data from several hundred women who have nursed their adopted babies. Most of them were referred to me for information and counseling (Hormann 1971; Hormann 1977).

Researchers who have actively sought out participants for their studies have a great many more than that. When Kathleen Auerbach and Jimmie Lynn Avery wanted to find out more about induced lactation and relactation, they heard from 606 respondents from the United States, Canada,

New Zealand, and the United Kingdom. Two hundred and forty of them were adoptive mothers. All of these contacts were made in a single year, suggesting that the figures might have been in the thousands had they been collected over several years (Auerbach 1981).

Avery, in her chapter, "Relactation and Induced Lactation" in *A Practical Guide to Breastfeeding* reported 2000 clients counseled over a six-year period in a Denver, Colorado relactation clinic and 1200 a year at a lactation clinic in southern California (Riordan 1983). While she doesn't distinguish between induced lactation and relactation in these figures, had the percentages been similar to those in her study with Auerbach (39.6 percent adoptive mothers) that one breastfeeding clinic in Southern California would have seen some 475 adoptive mothers every year.

During the last two decades of the Twentieth Century, there was an explosion of research on this topic and right at the end of the century the World Health Organization commissioned a literature review to explore the practice world-wide (Hormann and Savage 1998).

Myth 2: It is inappropriate.

But is breastfeeding an adopted baby appropriate just because it has become popular? Some people have argued that it is not. Linda Cannon Burgess, an adoption worker with many years experience in both placement and supervision, suggested in her book, *The Art of Adoption*, that an adoptive mother who wanted to breastfeed her baby was "completely off-base" and "creating a fiction by simulating natural motherhood and waiving the reality of adoption" (Burgess 1976). Avery also commented that for a long while "general public reaction was quite negative" to adoptive breastfeeding and it "was viewed as impossible, physiologically abnormal, and possibly perverse" (Riordan 1983). That perception is beginning to change now and many adoptive mothers are finding quite a lot of support in unexpected quarters (Baker 2002).

There is no scientific basis for these negative beliefs about adoptive breastfeeding. They are sheer speculation growing out of a psychological perspective that views any intimacy as the breeding ground for pathology. Kathryn Anderson (1986), commenting on critics who suggest that an adoptive mother who breastfeeds is trying to pretend that she gave birth to her baby, noted with exquisite good sense that "the sheer conscious effort of inducing lactation is so great that avoidance of reality would be impossible."

Consider, too, that a woman breastfeeding a baby she had not given birth to was, until very recently in human history, quite routine. This practice was often referred to as wet nursing. There are references to it in literature starting with the Bible. Moses, the most famous example, was actually breastfed by his own mother after being adopted by Pharaoh's daughter. But Obed (grandfather of King David), when he was born to Ruth and Boaz, was given to

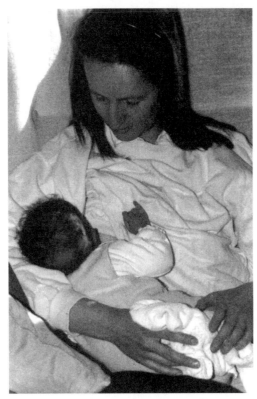

Breastfeeding your adopted baby is a tangible gift for both of you.

Ruth's former mother-in-law, "And Naomi took the child and laid him on her bosom, and became nurse to him" (King James Bible).

We don't know the name of the most memorable wet nurse in literature. The woman who breastfed Juliet is only called "Nurse" in "Romeo and Juliet". But we do know that she had had a daughter, Susan, who died and that the bond between her and her young charge, Juliet, was warm and tender.

It might be argued that in former times, breastfeeding was so important that wet nursing could be justified–but that it is no longer appropriate in developed countries. There is no support in practice or in the literature for the view that mother's milk is no longer very important or that breastfeeding a child you have not given birth to yourself is inherently pathological or somehow "unnatural."

Myth 3: It is impossible.

Traditionally, wet nurses have been women who have borne children and breastfed them alongside their hired nurslings. For these women, it was just a matter of continuing or increasing lactation that was already in progress. But that hasn't always been the case. Naomi's sons had grown up, married and had died some time before her daughter-in-law, Ruth, remarried and produced Obed. And Ruth is not the only grandmother reported to have induced lactation. One researcher described three cases of grandmothers or older women inducing lactation for orphaned infants. She also reported two cases at the other end of the spectrum in which, "a young girl who had never had a baby took a tiny motherless baby and nursed it at her breast, successfully stimulating a supply of nourishing fluid and rearing the mite." (Phillips 1969a).

In 1988 in Ethiopia, I was introduced to a woman who had relactated for her nine-month-old twin grandchildren after her daughter ran away. The physician who verified this experience had told her she would have to breastfeed the babies or they would die. So she did. She was not a young grandmother as we suppose some breastfeeding grandmothers to be. She pulled her breasts out of her dress for me to see and told me proudly "These old breasts were 56 years old when they made milk for my grandbabies."

Chapter 2
How Lactation Works

How is it possible for a woman who has not recently had a baby or has never had one to stimulate lactation? A little explanation of breast anatomy and the physiology of lactation may be helpful here.

Anatomy and physiology

The breasts are made up of a combination of glandular and adipose (fat) tissue. To a large extent, it is the fat that determines breast size and shape, but it is the glandular tissue that makes lactation possible.

Deep in the breasts are numerous alveoli, the fundamental units of the glandular system. They are made up of secretory cells, which make the milk, and myoepithelial cells, which contract to move the milk into small ductules. These ductules, like small branches of a tree, merge into larger mammary ducts, which carry the milk down to the nipple. The whole system is referred to as a lobe. Each breast has between 7 and 10 of these lobes or mini-milk factories. Ongoing research continues to reveal more details about the anatomy of the lactating breast (Hartmann 2002).

The breast is served by a large number of blood vessels, which usually become quite visible in pregnancy and lactation. Few women need to be told that there is also a high concentration of nerves in the breasts that makes them sensitive to pleasure and to pain. The dark pigmented area surrounding the nipple is called the areola. Small glands in the areola, the Montgomery glands, secrete a nipple lubricant that is also mildly antiseptic. The nipple itself has several small openings through which the milk can flow.

Hormonal influences

Virtually all women have developed a system of alveoli and ducts during puberty. Mammary growth is further stimulated by the cycle of ovulation and menstruation up to about age 35, but it is during pregnancy that the really dramatic changes, which prepare the breasts to feed the baby, occur. The alveoli grow larger under the influence of progesterone. Meanwhile, the system of ducts expands and specializes, thanks to estrogen. By the third month of pregnancy, the anterior pituitary gland (hypothalamus) has become involved, stimulating the release of prolactin, and colostrum begins to be produced. The expectant mother may notice this around the 16th week of pregnancy.

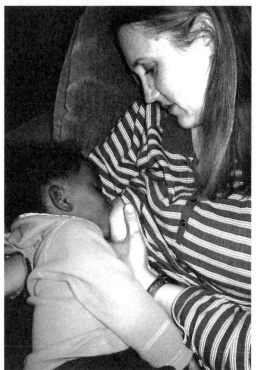

Once the baby is born, the hormonal balance shifts. Estrogen and progesterone decrease, prolactin increases. The hypothalamus signals the alveoli to start producing milk and these tiny cells take on the very complex job of making milk out of the nutrients and water they extract from the mother's bloodstream. They are at it continually, minute after minute, hour after hour, day after day for as long as the baby's suckling signals that milk is still needed.

Julianna resting peacefully at her adoptive mother's breast.

Lactation follows pregnancy quite automatically even after a late miscarriage, a stillbirth, or a neonatal death. The mother who does not put her baby to breast will still lactate for a while but continued lactation depends on frequent removal of milk from the breast. This is good news for the adoptive mother.

Regular, frequent breast stimulation acts as a signal to the pituitary to secrete the hormones prolactin and oxytocin. Prolactin is responsible for milk production; oxytocin controls the milk ejection or "let-down" reflex. Many adoptive mothers notice drops of milk in the early weeks of breastfeeding, on average around the fourth week, but it may be some time before there is a reasonable supply of milk. There is a good explanation for that.

Establishing a milk supply under normal conditions requires a very high level of prolactin. Prolactin rises gradually during pregnancy, drops just a few hours before birth, and then reaches new heights after the baby has suckled. The level remains high for the first week whether a mother puts her baby to breast or not. From the second week postpartum to about the 12th, baseline levels of prolactin are six to ten times those in a non-lactating woman. Those levels may double following suckling. Between six months and a year after birth, a breastfeeding mother's blood levels of prolactin decline to three to four times the levels in a non-lactating woman. Suckling continues to cause levels to double over the baseline through the second year.

The adoptive mother does not have the advantage of high prolactin levels to prime her lactational pump. Because milk production is controlled, to a certain extent, by prolactin, it will only happen if prolactin release is stimulated in response to suckling, pumping, and/or the use of galactagogues (natural or chemical substances that promote milk production). (See Chapter 4.)

Psychological and cultural factors

The experience in developed countries has been that milk production in adoptive mothers is likely to remain below the level needed for full lactation. Women in developing countries, however, tend to have better milk supplies under the same circumstances. It is reasonable to assume that some psycho-cultural factors are involved and a recent review of the literature strengthens that assumption (Gribble 2004).

The course of lactation

As the milk supply increases, the alveoli and ducts probably expand gradually as they do during pregnancy. Some women experience significant breast growth during the pre-ovulatory and immediate post-ovulatory phases of their menstrual cycles but this varies considerably from woman to woman. Some adoptive mothers may experience a variation in milk production connected to menstruation. Establishing lactation without benefit of an immediately preceding pregnancy depends primarily on frequent, effective breast stimulation. It takes longer to establish than it does after a pregnancy and the course may be very uneven.

Chapter 3

Preparing for Adoptive Breastfeeding

It is usually helpful to do some advance preparation if you are planning to breastfeed your adopted baby.

Psychological preparation and motivation

Psychological preparation is the first step. Why do you want to breastfeed your baby? What are you expecting the experience to be like? Who do you have to support you?

If you want to breastfeed your baby to enhance the closeness between you, to give him skin-to-skin contact, to help him with hand-eye coordination and good facial and jaw development, you are on the right track. Most of these things are possible with bottle-feeding, too, but they flow quite naturally from breastfeeding and breastfeeding can add a delightful dimension to your nurturing if your expectations are realistic.

But suppose you are thinking more about nutrition and allergy prevention, suppose the simplicity and ease of breastfeeding are the big attractions, or you doubt your ability to bond to a baby you haven't breastfed? Such expectations may make your experience with breastfeeding and/or adoption harder. Breastfeeding an adopted baby is neither simple nor easy. There is no guarantee of milk (though most mothers have some) and most

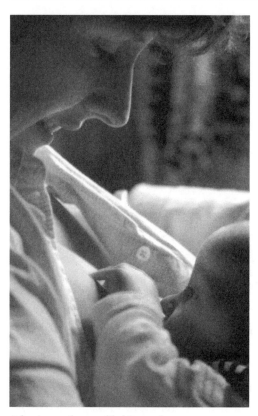

Adoptive mothers and babies need encouragement and accurate information.

importantly, your baby needs your love and your commitment to him regardless of how breastfeeding turns out.

Unrealistic expectations can turn an experience that is meant to promote bonding and security into one that is intolerably stressful for the whole family. A mother embarking on adoptive breastfeeding or relactation needs to be prepared for the possibility that she might not have a full milk supply or that her baby will not learn to breastfeed effectively. If she isn't prepared, her confidence in her ability to mother her baby may be severely undermined. Occasionally, when the mother has had her heart set on breastfeeding no matter what, the adoption has been disrupted when her breastfeeding relationship with her baby failed to live up to her expectations.

Breastfeeding is a wonderful option for many adoptive mothers and their babies, but it does require far more patience and commitment than breastfeeding a homegrown baby. It is not suitable for families in which the mother or the baby is so stressed by learning to breastfeed that bonding and the sheer enjoyment of each other is compromised. Bottle-feeding—always in arms—is a much better choice for these families.

Breast stimulation by hand

If you have some time before your baby is due to arrive, you may want to do some breast stimulation in advance. The simplest method is hand expression because you need no equipment but your breasts and your hands. The idea is to stimulate all the milk ducts around the circumference of the areola on a frequent, regular schedule.

One method is to cup the breast in your hand with the thumb above and the first two fingers below, an inch to an inch and a half (2.5 to 4 cm) behind your nipple. Push back toward the chest wall while exerting gentle pressure on the milk ducts beneath your fingers. Rotate your hand around your breast to reach all the milk ducts. Switch hands halfway through or you will find your elbow in an impossibly awkward position. Express for three to five minutes before you switch to the other breast. If you have time, repeat the process on each breast to provide especially good stimulation. The whole procedure should take about 20 minutes.

The Marmet Technique of Manual Expression combines breast massage and stroking with an especially gentle and effective way of expressing. It is described in full in the Appendix.

Some mothers increase the effectiveness of hand expression with additional techniques that encourage blood flow to the breast and release of prolactin and oxytocin. A back rub between your shoulder blades (where the nerves to the breast radiate) is relaxing and encourages circulation to the breasts. One technique is especially good for encouraging the let-down reflex. Sit at a table with your head resting on your arms, your breasts hanging loose. Your back-rubber should stand behind you and using the knuckles of both hands move briskly along both sides of the spine from the base of your neck to below your shoulder blades. This can be repeated a few times and/or combined with a more extensive back and shoulder massage before pumping (WHO 1993).

Some mothers have found another technique effective for priming the pump. Using the palms of your hand or your fingertips, rub your nipples briskly but gently for a few minutes. The nipples should become erect and may tingle a bit after you have done this. With practice it should take less than a minute to get your nipples erect. Some couples consciously increase breast stimulation in their lovemaking when they are waiting for an adopted baby. The fathers in these couples often welcome the chance this gives them to help prepare for their new babies.

Whatever techniques of massage and hand expression you choose, they are most effective done at regular intervals—ideally every two or three hours during the day with a longer interval at night—much the same schedule you would hope for with a newborn baby. Realistically, this schedule may be impractical especially if you are working or have young children already. (Breastfeeding every two or three hours is a lot easier than pumping or expressing that often.) Hand expressing two or three times a day—morning and evening when you are undressed anyway and perhaps one other time—may still be helpful in developing the alveoli and ducts in your breasts.

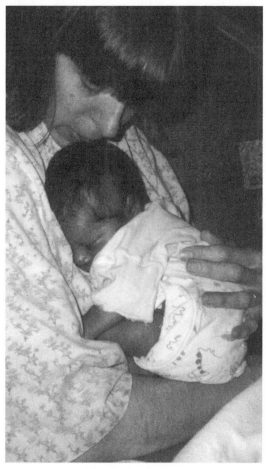

A mother's relationship with her child is precious.

How do you know it is helping? Possibly you won't, but there may be some signs in your breasts. They might become larger or feel firmer. Perhaps you will notice some tenderness or a sense of fullness in your breasts—or your nipples will protrude more. Drops of colostrum or milk are one sure sign that something is happening and many women see that evidence within the first six weeks of pumping. If you are not among them, don't lose heart. Even fully lactating women sometimes have difficulty with expressing milk. It is a learned skill that has no relationship to how well a baby will suckle or how much mother and baby will enjoy the breastfeeding relationship.

Breast stimulation with a pump

Some women prefer a portable or electric pump to hand expression and many women switch to one of these once they are getting some drops of colostrum or milk with hand expression.

Both sorts of pumps provide good rhythmic stimulation. Many of them have suction regulators that allow you to choose a comfortable setting. An electric model that pumps both breasts simultaneously gives especially good stimulation. Some electric models leave the mother's hands free and that can be a great relief. The drawbacks to these are that they can be cumbersome and expensive (though some models are quite reasonably priced) and they may not be as effective in stimulating prolactin secretion as hand expression. Pumps are, after all, machines, and many women, no matter how hard they try to visualize a baby at the breast, have a harder time responding to the pump than they do to their partner's touch or their own hands.

Avery suggested a possible psychological risk associated with pumping. "I have found that using the breast pump focuses the mother's attention on the milk rather than on bonding" (Riordan 1983).

With adoptive breastfeeding, keeping the nurturing and the natural desire to nourish the baby at the breast in proper balance is a challenge. Prepare for your baby in ways that are comfortable and effective for you. Milk supply is of interest, but mothering is paramount.

Chapter 4

Galactogogues: Substances that Help Start Milk Production

There has long been interest in a magic potion or pill that would stimulate or enhance milk production. Lawrence noted that, "Some medications that have been tried in relactation seem only to work when the breast has been primed by mammogenesis (that is by pregnancy)" (Lawrence 2005). In recent years, however, there has been some promising work with galactogogues even among women who have never been pregnant. Some of these are discussed in the sections that follow.

Herbs

Almost every culture has its favorite herbs for stimulating milk production. They haven't been studied enough to say that one or the other is **the** herb for making milk, but there is some intriguing experience. Paul Fleiss, in an article on herbs and the breastfeeding mother, mentioned no fewer than three dozen herbs that have been used to stimulate milk production, the most successful of which appears to have been fenugreek (Fleiss 1988). A recent review of galactogogues cites some 1200 anecdotal reports of using fenugreek resulting in an increase in milk production within 24 to 72 hours after starting it (Gabay 2002). However, there have not been any controlled trials on its use in promoting lactation. Diana West includes an interesting discussion of herbal galactogogues in her book, DEFINING YOUR OWN SUCCESS: BREASTFEEDING AFTER BREAST REDUCTION SURGERY. Sheila Humphrey's book, *A Nursing Mother's Herbal,* also provides information.

Hormones

Synthetic hormones have also been tried in varying combinations. Most commonly, mothers report using estrogen, progesterone, thyroid, and oxytocin (usually in the form of a nasal spray) to stimulate or increase the milk supply.

Twenty-two of the 65 women in my 1977 study—just over a third—reported using some sort of hormonal preparation prior to getting a baby and they were no more successful at producing milk than were the two-thirds who didn't use hormones (Hormann 1977). Half of the women in the Auerbach and Avery study on relactation used a synthetic oxytocin spray to enhance the milk-ejection reflex. Other hormones were rarely used. All of the mothers in this study were relactating for their biological infants and there was no indication given that they produced

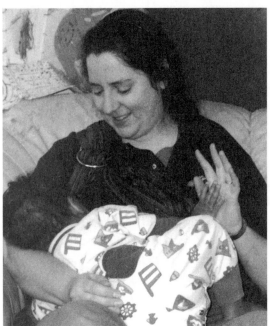

Pamela Willett with 11-month-old Orion.

more milk than the mothers not using oxytocin. (Auerbach and Avery 1980).

Case studies are being collected at present on a Canadian protocol involving continuous use of a combination birth control pill (1 mg progesterone, >0.035 mg estrogen for the regular protocol; 2 mg progesterone, >0.035 mg estrogen for the accelerated and menopause versions) along with domperidone for several weeks or months prior to beginning breastfeeding. Four to six weeks before the expected arrival of the baby, the birth control pill is stopped. Breast stimulation and the herbs, fenugreek (trigonella foenum-graecum) and blessed thistle (cnicus benedictus), are added to the domperidone. A change to the original accelerated and menopausal version of the protocol was based on new data indicating a four-fold increased risk of deep vein thrombosis with the dosages previously recommended. Initial reports on the protocol are promising in terms of milk production, but results are preliminary at this point (www.asklenore.info).

Using birth control pills uninterruptedly in this way may not be acceptable to many women no matter how eager they are to produce milk. The risks associated with synthetic hormones are well documented (EMEA 2001).

To date there have been no controlled studies that would definitely prove or disprove an overwhelming advantage to hormone therapy in establishing lactation, increasing milk supply, or stimulating the milk ejection reflex. On the whole, adoptive mothers are not relying on a hormonal boost to get lactation started.

Medications

Tranquillizing drugs have also long been part of the galactogogue repertoire. The occasional beer or glass of wine has, in the past, been suggested to help a tense mother relax and increase her milk production. Today we know that alcohol intake "decreases prolactin yield, blocks release of oxytocin, and can inhibit the milk ejection reflex" (Riordan and Auerbach 1999). Lawrence (2005) notes that "alcohol blocks the release of oxytocin" and "[T]he impact of alcohol on oxytocin is dose related." Schaefer (2005) observes, "Occasional, limited use of alcohol" (once or twice a week) "is no impediment to breastfeeding." Both Lawrence and Dr. Tom Hale suggest avoiding breastfeeding for at least two (2) hours after drinking alcohol (Hale 2006).

Among the drugs most often used to induce lactation are chlorpromazine (an anti-psychotic) and two peristaltic stimulators, metoclopramide and domperidone. All of these drugs increase prolactin secretion.

Derrick Jelliffe first reported using chlorpromazine in his relactation clinics in Uganda (Jelliffe and Jelliffe 1978). Karen Pryor described his method in an early edition of *Nursing Your Baby*.

"He puts the mothers to bed (with their babies, of course) to provide adequate rest. He takes the bottle away. . . . He orders the mother to nurse her baby every two hours. He gives the mother plenty of milk to drink both to keep her fluid intake up and to suggest that what goes in must come out ('sympathetic magic'). He gives her a therapeutic dose of chlorpromazine (100 mg three times daily), which may or may not have an effect on lactation. . . . For the first day or two, he also administers an oxytocin nasal spray just before each feeding. The mother usually finds that by the third day of Dr. Jelliffe's regimen she has ample milk once more." (Pryor 1973)

These women and the women reported in Brown's review of relactation in refugee camps were, for the most part, relactating for their own, very young babies. However, some of the women in Brown's report had been hired to induce lactation. Once a milk supply had been established, the study planned for each woman to provide milk for two orphaned babies (Brown 1978).

Some of the more recent research in this area is also quite intriguing. Banapurmath (India) and Nemba (Papua New Guinea) published their prospective studies with adoptive mothers in 1993 and 1994. Banapurmath's research involved relactation. All ten mothers in the study had at one time or another experienced pregnancy and childbirth. There was a lactation gap of between one and 16 years. The adopted babies were between eight days and five months of age. Two mothers—those who had not breastfed for six and for sixteen years—were able to breastfeed their babies exclusively within about six weeks. Three additional mothers were able to breastfeed their children partially within two to four weeks. The other mothers gave up the attempt after two weeks (Banapurmath 1993b).

Even more impressive was Nemba's study of 37 women of whom 12 had never before lactated. Among the 25 who had breastfed before, the lactation gap ranged from four months to 21 years. The children were similar in age to those in the Indian study—five days to five months. In this study as well, some women gave up the attempt early. Nineteen women with prior experience of breastfeeding and 11 without it remained. In the first group, three pairs were eliminated: one infant died; two were returned to the biological mother. Altogether, 16 women with prior breastfeeding experience attempted to breastfeed their adoptive or foster infants. Thirteen of them had adequate milk production within five to 10 days after starting chlorpromazine or metoclopramide and breastfed altogether at least nine months. If milk production is viewed as success, 81 percent of these mothers were successful. Eleven of the 12 mothers (92 percent) with no prior breastfeeding experience were able to provide their babies with sufficient milk within five to 13 days after starting chlorpromazine or metoclopramide.

How did they achieve these astounding results? The studies reported that over the first 10 to 15 days, the Indian mothers were given 10 mg of metoclopramide three times a day. Mothers in Papua, New Guinea, received either the same or 25 mg of chlorpromazine four times a day. Some women who had never lactated before received both drugs. In the second study (Nemba), the women without prior breastfeeding experience had a one-time injection of 100 mg Depo-Provera (medroxyprogesterone) a week before they began taking the metoclopramide or chlorpromazine. Galactogogues may have played a role. But are they necessary? Another Banapurmath study on relactation—mostly by the mothers who had given birth to the babies—did not involve galactogogues and had nearly the same results. This suggests that while galactogogues may sometimes be useful, they are not essential to a good milk supply (Banapurmath 1993a).

These studies highlight essential factors. In one of Banapurmath's studies (1993b), the infants had been admitted to the hospital because of serious illness. The mothers in Nemba's study were all adopting or fostering infants. Induced lactation or relactation was attempted on physician's orders and was supported with comprehensive counseling and regular checkups. A breastfeeding frequency of eight to 12 times a day was prescribed.

Of central importance is that these studies took place in countries in which breastfeeding is the cultural norm, where mothers can generally count on adequate **support** from their health care providers, their families, and the community. Indispensable as well for milk production, with or without galactogogues, is **good breastfeeding management**. This involves proper positioning and attachment to the breast, very frequent breastfeeding day and night, and feeds of sufficient length that 80 percent of the mother's milk is removed from the breasts to signal the need to produce more. So while galactogogues sometimes play a supporting role, good breastfeeding management and support are the crucial factors in both induced lactation and relactation.

Despite the exciting possibilities in using galactogogues, it must be emphasized that like hormone therapy, other drug therapy has drawbacks. Chlorpromazine is a powerful anti-psychotic. At relatively high levels (100 mg three times a day), it makes mothers drowsy (Brown 1978). Involuntary jerking motions have also been reported (Schaefer 2001; Hale 2006). In lower doses, it seems to have fewer side effects and may still be effective as a galactogogue. But where other drugs less likely to cause symptoms are available, using anti-psychotic drugs to enhance milk production may pose a risk that is unacceptably high for most mothers and their babies.

Metoclopramide is currently considered the drug of choice for breastfeeding mothers in Europe since it is the best studied (Schaefer 2001). Because only small amounts—less than the therapeutic dosage for an infant—are secreted into the milk, it does not pose any apparent risk to the baby. However, long-term use (more than four weeks) may be associated with maternal depression (Hale 2006).

Domperidone is the newest drug in the galactogogue repertoire. Like metoclopramide, it increases the flow of prolactin and may, thus, enhance milk production (Schaefer 2001). The Newman-Goldfarb protocol mentioned above involves prolonged use of domperidone starting several months before the estimated arrival of the baby and continuing throughout the breastfeeding period as well. The single controlled double-blind study of domperidone, involving mothers of premature infants, indicates a 28 percent average increase in milk production (Da Silva et al. 2001).

Unlike metoclopramide, domperidone does not cross the blood-brain barrier and its high molecular weight and protein binding do not allow significant transfer into the milk (Schaefer, personal communication). It might be a good alternative to metoclopramide where it is available; it is not currently available in the United States. Recent interventions and an Import Alert from the Federal Drug Administration (FDA) have limited the possibility of having it compounded in US pharmacies or importing it from another country (FDA 2004).

Special foods

Nearly every culture has some favorite foods or beverages thought to enhance milk production. The 1999 edition of Riordan and Auerbach

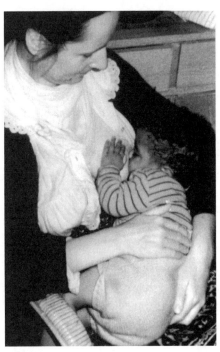

Márta Guóth-Gumberger with Peter during his second year of life.

included a guide to regional and ethnic foods believed to act as galactogogues. However, there is currently no scientific evidence to support the contention that particular foods or the mother's overall nutritional status affect either her ability to lactate adequately or, with one or two exceptions, the composition of the milk. On the contrary, the research clearly indicates that even a moderately malnourished woman can produce sufficient milk of good quality for her baby (Prentice 1988; National Academy of Sciences 1991).

Nevertheless, good maternal nutrition is important for all breastfeeding women—including those inducing lactation—because it ensures that the mother's own nutritional stores do not get depleted while she is breastfeeding her baby.

Since lactation requires considerable energy (more so than pregnancy), the World Health Organization (WHO) recommends that breastfeeding mothers take in an additional 325 to 425 calories per day (Michaelsen et al. 2000). The European WHO Office suggests a diet for both pregnant and breastfeeding mothers that includes:

- 6 to11 portions of bread, cereals, pasta, rice, or potato
- 5 portions (for a total of 400 g) vegetables and fruit
- 3 portions milk or other dairy products
- 2 portions fish, poultry, meat or beans
- Minimal fat, sugar, and salt
- Folic acid and iron supplements for mothers at risk of deficiencies

Among food supplements, brewer's yeast (nutritional, not baker's yeast) is popular—not for its taste—as an enhancement to milk production among many breastfeeding mothers in the United States (Black et al. 1998). Its high B-vitamin content may actually be helpful in soothing frayed nerves and indirectly boosting milk production, but at this point, there is only anecdotal evidence for its potential to increase milk production.

Herbal teas with some combination of fennel, coriander, chamomile, borage, blessed thistle, lemongrass, comfrey, anise, and/or fenugreek are widely used as galactogogues in Europe, but are not well studied.

It isn't necessary to make heroic efforts to put together just the right diet. It is enough to have a generally well-balanced diet with a reasonable amount of fluid. Too much fluid can actually decrease your milk supply; so don't force yourself to drink more than you really want to (Duisdieker et al. 1985).

As you consider all the suggestions in chapters 3 and 4, remember that your baby is the *sine qua non* in induced lactation. He is what the preparation is all about. If you didn't have any time to prepare (many babies arrive with practically no notice), don't worry about it. Many of the happiest adoptive breastfeeding experiences have been with babies whose arrivals took their mothers by surprise.

Chapter 5

Beginning Breastfeeding with Your Adopted Baby

Holding your baby

With or without preparation, the moment will come when you have your baby and wonder: "How do I start?" The easiest way to begin is to put your baby to your breast and see what happens. If you have breastfed before you will know how it is done, but your baby may need some time to learn how. If this is your first baby—or the first you have breastfed—both you and your baby will be amateurs and you will need to be patient while both of you figure out what to do.

The Womanly Art of Breastfeeding has good photo illustrations for positioning your baby at the breast (LLLI 2004). You might also take a look at *Bestfeeding: Getting Breastfeeding Right for You,* which has a step-by-step illustrated guide through the process (Renfrew et al. 2000).

You will probably want to begin with the traditional cradle hold, with your baby tummy to tummy facing you. His head should be positioned comfortably on your arm so he doesn't have to stretch to reach the breast. Tickle his lips lightly with your nipple in case he hasn't already opened his mouth and started rooting around for the breast. When his mouth is open wide, at about a 120° angle, move him onto the breast.

Some babies open their mouths only a little bit at first. If your baby is one of these, wait a minute and then tickle his lips again. He will open his mouth wider as he gets more eager to find the breast.

Check with your hand that he has his lower jaw over the lower part of your areola. His lips should not be rolled inward as he suckles. You can pull his lower lip down gently to check that his tongue is correctly positioned, under the breast and stretched right out to the gum line.

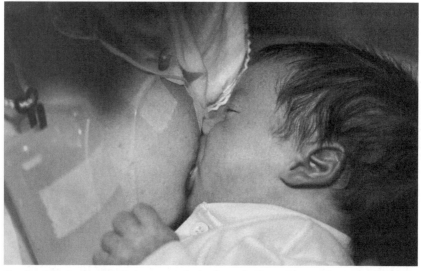

Good positioning is critically important during breastfeeding, with or without supplementing: the baby's mouth is wide open; he has grasped the areola and both lips are rolled outwards.

It is all much easier than it sounds and takes less time to accomplish than to read about. Most mother and baby pairs figure it out quite naturally, but if you want to reassure yourself that you are doing it right or you are not quite sure about it, you will need to know what you are looking for.

Breastfeeding frequency

Offer your baby lots of opportunities at your breast—at least every two or three hours in the daytime and during the night with one longer break—up to four or five hours—if he is sleeping of his own accord. Let him suckle as long as he wants. If he is positioned properly, you probably won't have any trouble with sore nipples. If you do, recheck the position of his mouth. Any initial soreness should fade gradually. If soreness becomes worse, seek help from an experienced breastfeeding counselor.

Part of the reason for breastfeeding frequently is to stimulate your milk supply. Most babies want to breastfeed very often and most mothers need that frequent stimulation to get breastfeeding firmly established. This rhythm usually meshes nicely with the baby's needs. If he is getting mother's milk he will probably be hungry every couple of hours and even if he is getting a substitute, the frequent skin contact is important for his emotional and physical well-being. Gently encourage your baby to go to the breast for comfort and to fall asleep. Even if the bulk of his nutrition is coming from other sources, his nurturing can come primarily from you.

Helping your baby feel comfortable at the breast

Sometimes parents worry that it may confuse or frustrate the baby if he is offered the breast when the mother is not fully lactating. This same question is never posed with regard to a pacifier or the baby's thumb. The baby doesn't expect milk from either of them. He sucks for the sheer delight of it and when he is hungry, he lets his mother know. He can just as well comfort himself at his mother's breast and it is even better because his mother, with all her soothing sounds and wonderful smells, is right there as he sucks. It is really much nicer than sucking his thumb or a pacifier somewhere away from her. Even if you never produce a drop of milk, the baby who has learned to suck for comfort at your breast will not be disappointed. He does not expect it any more than the breastfeeding baby born to his mother expects her breasts to be overflowing with milk all the time. This baby also sucks for comfort when he is not interested in feeding.

Very young babies usually take quite easily to the breast even if they have already had some experience with bottles. It will be easier for both you and your baby if you can plan the first few breastfeeding sessions for times when he is not famished or overtired and in a place where you can sit comfortably and have some privacy. If he is not keen on it at first, don't give up and don't take it personally. Babies need time to learn new skills or to warm up to new ideas. We recognize this when we introduce them to a cup or a spoon, for instance, and we don't stop trying because they turn their heads away or make a terrible fuss the first few times. Mothers who are weaning their babies from breast to bottle don't feel hurt or insulted if their babies reject the bottle at first. They know that changes take some getting used to.

Mothers weaning the baby from bottle to breast know this too, but they may feel hurt and rejected just the same when their babies refuse the breast. A little perspective and patience are important here. Your adopted baby is being asked to bond to a new mother and learn a new way of sucking. If he resists, it doesn't mean he doesn't like you or that he will never learn. He needs to adjust to the changes in his life and he needs your love, commitment, and gentle encouragement while he is doing it.

Sometimes a baby learns to breastfeed in stages, first accustoming himself to the feel of his mother's skin as he bottle-feeds, then gradually lying contentedly against her breast without the bottle. If the mother is patient and relaxed, he will eventually explore the breast—as he does every new object—with his mouth. Often a baby will suckle at the breast more readily when he is sleepy. After practicing in his sleep for a while, he will very likely be ready to breastfeed when he is awake. The mother of an adopted newborn has a very good chance of establishing a breastfeeding relationship with her baby even if he is not fully—or even partially—fed on mother's milk.

Breastfeeding the older baby

Many babies don't join their families as newborns. For one reason or another, placement is delayed for several weeks or months. Is there any chance of breastfeeding these babies? We used to think that babies over three or four

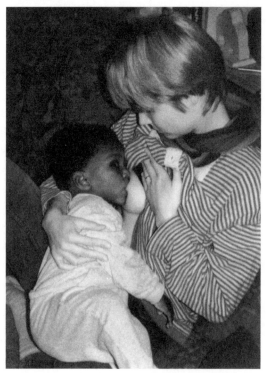

Corinna Männchen breastfeeds Emmanuel. He was about a year old when he came to his adoptive family.

months probably could not be taught to breastfeed. But the experience of adoptive mothers has frequently contradicted
that assumption.

One baby in my experience began nursing at seven-and-a-half months and took quite happily to the breast (Morris, personal communication). Another baby, adopted at a year, needed several weeks before she was comfortable even being touched (Holohan 1983). The mother had abandoned all thought of breastfeeding her because of her age, but the baby had other ideas. After observing an older sibling at the breast, she indicated she wanted to breastfeed as well and continued for many months. Yet another mother reported to me that she began breastfeeding her adopted baby at 17 months. She suspected he had been breastfed by his foster mother in Korea so he may not have been such a late learner after all. Older babies who resist the breast at first can sometimes learn to suck at the breast, but it takes patience and systematic training (Guoth-Gumberger 1994).

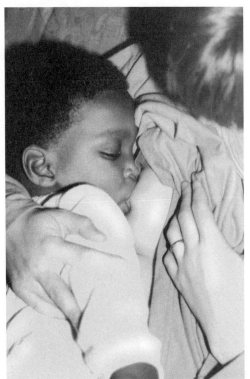

No one can say for certain whether a particular baby is too old to learn to breastfeed. If your baby is older and you would like to breastfeed—just try it and see what happens. Like mothers of newborns, mothers trying to breastfeed older adopted babies need to be patient with their babies and with themselves. They have to be creative in devising ways to get their babies in touch with them and they need to keep an open mind because the **baby's** mind may really be made up. At any age, breastfeeding is only part of a

Emmanuel, a little older.

whole range of skin-to-skin and heart-to-heart experiences that draw a mother and her baby close and keep them close. If breastfeeding your adopted baby becomes an end in itself, the situation could become too stressful to promote the kind of bond you want to foster between you.

Chapter 6

Supplements

Virtually all adopted babies will need some supplementary nourishment. At the beginning, the baby may be getting all his nourishment from a source other than his mother's milk, but in the context of adoptive breastfeeding, that is still called "supplementation."

Choosing a supplement

You will likely want to talk to your pediatrician about the kind of supplement to use. It will depend on many factors: what your baby has been getting thus far, his health, any allergies he may have, and, to some extent, your own preference.

While nothing really comes close to mother's milk, modern, fully adapted formulas are the most adequate nutritionally. Follow the instructions for preparation carefully and pay close attention to hygiene. Because no powdered formula is sterile, it should always be made up with water that has been boiled and cooled off to about 158° F (70° C) or use the (sterile) liquid concentrate and mix with boiled, cool water.

If your baby is unable to tolerate any kind of artificial baby milk—and this is very unlikely—there are, in many countries, milk banks, which will provide human milk on prescription. (See milk bank information in the Resources.)

Deciding how much supplement to offer

It is important to give your baby enough supplement to nourish him well. Your own observations will let you know if he is getting enough. He should have at least six very wet diapers a day. If he is getting enough fluid, the urine will be pale or colorless. Bowel activity will vary from baby to baby and from week to week with the same baby. He may have a stool with every feeding or it may be less frequently. A normal stool is soft. The formula-fed baby's stool will be more formed than a breastfed baby's stool. Many babies strain and appear quite uncomfortable when they are having a bowel movement. That does not mean they are constipated. Texture tells a lot more than timing.

A well-nourished baby will also be gaining weight—about four to six ounces (115 to 180 g) a week in the first four months on average is fine— but you probably won't need a scale to tell. Your baby will feel heavier, his legs and arms will fill out, and he will outgrow his clothes. A well-nourished baby will have the energy for other developmental tasks as well. He will practice holding up his head, he will learn to smile, to respond to your voice, and to turn over. With a little practice, your observations can tell you very well if he is growing and developing as he should be. Usually your regularly scheduled doctor's examination and weight check of your baby will only confirm what you already know.

You may have heard that the supplement should be restricted or watered down to encourage the baby to work harder at the breast. This used to be suggested sometimes, but with experience, it became clear that this was not in the baby's best interest. Underfeeding can have long-term consequences for the baby's overall growth and for brain development. Make sure your baby gets all he needs to eat. You can manage the breastfeeding so that he still has plenty of time at the breast even if his nutrition is coming from another source.

Using a bottle

Perhaps the most common way to feed an adoptive baby is by using a bottle. Bottles are familiar in developed countries, so parents are likely to know how to use them. They almost always have markings on the side so it is easy to measure how much the baby is drinking. But the baby who sucks at a bottle may have difficulty learning to suckle at the breast or he may satisfy his sucking needs at the bottle. For this reason, many adoptive breastfeeding mothers limit the use of bottles and feed the supplement in another way.

Using a cup

Even very young babies can be successfully fed by cup. The World Health Organization (WHO) and The United Nations Children's Fund (UNICEF) recommend this method for babies in developing countries who are not able to feed directly at their mothers' breasts or who temporarily need supplements (Lang 1994). Some hospitals—even in developed countries—have completely eliminated bottles and give supplements only by cup (BFHI News 1999).

There are two reasons for this recommendation. One is that bottles are more difficult to keep clean. In developing countries, lack of clean water, fuel, and soap often make it impossible. This reason is usually not as significant in developed countries when careful attention is paid to hygiene. However, the other risk with bottle-feeding—that your baby will have trouble learning to suck effectively at the breast—is equally important anywhere in the world. When you use a cup to feed your baby, you can keep track of how much he is taking by measuring the amount of supplement before and after feeding. Some hospitals use simple plastic cups to feed. You may find it more convenient to use a shot glass or a small (2 oz or 50 ml) plastic or paper cup. Until you get used to it, protect your baby and yourself from spills with a large terry cloth towel. Using a cup to feed your baby may seem unusual to you at first, but to a newborn baby, it's just another skill to learn. Most babies learn quickly.

Using a syringe

Some parents prefer to have their babies associate sucking with feeding and for these families there are a couple of possibilities to choose from. A syringe with a soft attachment can be used to give the supplement (Walker 1991). Place your (very clean) finger in your baby's mouth along with the syringe. When the baby sucks, push the plunger gently to deliver a little milk. As his sucking is reinforced with food, he will continue to suck until he is no longer hungry. It is an easy technique to learn and most babies can finish four oz (100 ml) or so in 20 or 30 minutes, hardly longer than the average breast or bottle-feeding.

Using a nursing supplementer

A nursing supplementer is a specialized version of the syringe technique with an important difference. Milk is delivered at the breast as the baby feeds—and the baby controls the flow. In the past, some mothers used a small pipette, an eyedropper, or a syringe to drip milk into their babies' mouths while they were breastfeeding. Today many mothers prefer to use a specially designed at-breast nursing supplementer. With the nursing supplementer, the baby stimulates the breast every time he feeds and he associates breastfeeding with eating. These devices have become very popular with adoptive mothers.

The original nursing supplementer, the Lact-Aid, was designed by an adoptive father when his wife was breastfeeding their baby (Avery 1998). A small disposable plastic bag—similar to the inserts in some bottle systems— is used to hold the supplement. A hard plastic plug keeps the bag closed. Joined to the plug is a fine tube that is positioned near the mother's nipple when the baby is at the breast. As the baby suckles, the supplement is

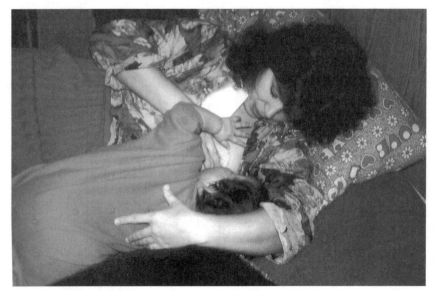

Elena Iskraut breastfeeding Emmanuel using a nursing supplementer.

released. A cord attached to the supplementer allows the mother to wear it around her neck or attach it to her bra. By adjusting the position of the bag, the amount of effort the baby needs to make to get the milk can also be adjusted.

Other nursing supplementers have a different design. Medela's Supplemental Nursing System (SNS), for instance, uses two tubes and a hard plastic, rectangular bottle. It is a little harder to nurse discreetly with the SNS, but it is easier to change from side to side. A comprehensive, illustrated parent guide to using at-breast nursing supplementers has recently been published (Guóth-Gumberger 2006).

All nursing supplementers work on the same general principle. They are, in essence, artificial external reservoirs to hold the supplement and allow the baby to be fed **at** the breast if not fully **from** it.

Suggestions for Breastfeeding Management after the Early Phase

Because every baby is different, no schedule or breastfeeding plan will fit everybody, but there are a few things to keep in mind as you breastfeed your adopted baby.

Offer your baby the breast very frequently—at least every two or three hours during the day with one longer interval at night.

Your baby is more likely to suckle at the breast if he is not frantic with hunger. Try waking him up before you expect him to be hungry and let him suckle for a while before you offer him the supplement using a nursing supplementer, syringe, cup, eyedropper, or a bottle.

Give him a chance to stay at the breast after he has finished feeding. This is especially important if he is supplemented by cup or syringe because he cannot fulfill his sucking needs with these feeding methods. If you are using a bottle, remove it when he seems to have satisfied his hunger and put him to your breast for more suckling practice.

Avoid pacifiers as much as possible. The baby who uses a pacifier regularly is not going to suckle well at his mother's breast—even if she has a good milk supply. Help him learn from the beginning that his sucking needs are best met in your arms at your breast.

Encourage your baby to fall asleep at your breast. Most babies don't want to fall asleep alone in any case and there is no great advantage to a baby's learning to fall asleep on his own at an early age: Linking breastfeeding and falling asleep is one good way of ensuring that you will have a baby at your breast even if you aren't producing much milk.

Offer the breast between feeds whenever your baby seems fussy or discontented.

Using both breasts at each feed provides particularly good stimulation and helps develop your baby's hand-eye coordination.

Chapter 7

Reducing the Supplement/ Increasing Your Milk

Once your baby is feeding well at the breast and you have a bit of milk, you will probably start wondering how to know when to start cutting down on the supplement.

Guidelines for reducing the supplement

If your baby is using a nursing supplementer, a little milk left in it when he is finished feeding may be a signal that you could reduce the supplement. He might also refuse the last bit in his bottle, cup, or syringe. On the other hand, he might not. Then you will have to rely on your own observations of your baby and your good judgment.

You can safely reduce the formula in small increments. Some parents are most comfortable reducing the total supplement for the day by about half an ounce (15 ml) each day. Other families prefer to reduce the supplement amount at **each feeding** by the same amount for one 24-hour period and then maintain that level for several days while they see how the baby reacts and gains weight. In either case, the reductions would amount to about approximately four ounces (105 to 120 ml) a week.

As long as your baby continues to gain weight on this regime, the reductions can continue, but if his weight plateaus or slows down too much, that's a signal to stop reducing the supplement for a while or even to increase the amount of supplement for a while Every baby is different. Consider these factors when deciding about decreasing the amount of supplement you offer:

- Your baby's age and general health.
- Whether your baby is experiencing a growth spurt.
- Your general health.
- Whether your milk supply has started increasing.
- Family circumstances (avoid making drastic feeding changes when your family is under stress from a move, a family celebration, or other life changing event).

Regular weight checks (every two or three days) on an accurate scale are important during the time when you are reducing the amount of supplement you offer.

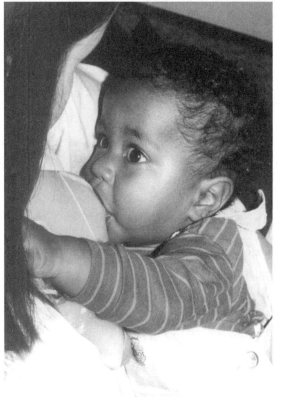

Your baby's adoring gaze makes it all worthwhile.

In between, keep track of how many diapers your baby uses and the consistency of your baby's bowel movements. (Placing a chart near where you usually change your baby can help you and other family members keep an accurate record.) Your baby should continue to have about as many wet and dirty diapers per day as he did before you started reducing the supplement.

Young babies who are exclusively formula-fed have light or dark brown bowel movements a couple of times

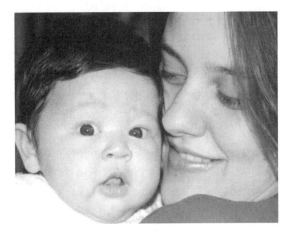

a day. Young exclusively breastfed babies have bowel movements that are about the consistency of cottage cheese and are usually bright yellow. They may have three to five movements a day. As your body starts making more milk, your baby's bowel movements will begin to change to be more like those of an exclusively breastfed baby. The older breastfed baby will have fewer bowel movements per day, but they will be bigger.

If your baby is more than six weeks old when he starts to learn to breast-feed, he will be more likely to have less frequent, larger bowel movements. However, as he begins to receive your milk, their color and consistency will change in a similar way to a younger baby's until the time when he starts eating complementary solid foods. Then the color and consistency will be darker and firmer once again.

Your baby's growth spurts

Growth spurts commonly occur at six weeks and three months, but there is wide variation. Your baby's appetite will suddenly increase and despite breastfeeding more frequently, you may have to postpone cutting back on the supplement or perhaps even increase it a little. Don't get discouraged by this. You will still be feeding less of the supplement than you would have been if you were not breastfeeding. Your milk supply is really still increasing, but so are your baby's needs.

Menstrual cycles and milk production

Menstrual cycles change the balance of hormones in your body and may affect your milk supply (LLLI 2004). Shortly before your period, your breasts may feel full, firm, and painfully tender to the touch. You may feel moody and notice that your milk supply seems lower or the let-down takes longer.

Should you experience this–and not every woman does–things will probably be back to normal within two or three days after your period starts and you'll begin to notice your supply increasing again.

Avery speculated that "the reduction in estrogen and progesterone that occurs at the onset of menses (is) similar in effect to the sharp drop in these hormones that occurs at birth when the placenta is expelled" and wonders if "the sudden postmenstrual increase in lactation (is) related to an increase in prolactin secretion during the secretory phase of menstruation" (Riordan 1983). There has been no research on this question, but it is worth noting that many adoptive mothers have reported a slow-down in lactation coinciding with the immediate premenstrual phase of their cycles. And non-adoptive breastfeeding mothers often notice similar effects on breastfeeding when their menstrual cycles resume.

Questions about exclusive breastfeeding

Q. Is it realistic to expect that a woman inducing lactation can fully breastfeed her baby?

A. One mother in my 1977 study—a woman who had previously lactated—was able to achieve a full milk supply. Auerbach and Avery (1981) reported on 240 adoptive mothers. Eighty-three had never been pregnant nor lactated; 55 had been pregnant but had never lactated; 102 had given birth and breastfed one or more babies. Of this latter group, 18 were still breastfeeding when they adopted. Nearly three-quarters (74%) of the mothers who had never been pregnant needed to supplement for the entire breastfeeding period. Slightly fewer (72%) of the women who had

Breastfeeding can be a very intense kind of communication between mother and child.

previously been pregnant, but had not lactated, supplemented until breast-feeding ended. Just over half (53%) of the mothers with prior breastfeeding experience supplemented throughout the time they were breastfeeding their adopted infants. Even among tandem nursing mothers, 39% continued to supplement. On the other hand, the studies from India and Papua-New Guinea mentioned above appear to demonstrate quite clearly that it is possible for adoptive mothers—even those who have not previously breastfed—to breastfeed their adoptive infants completely (Banapurmath 1993b; Nemba 1994). However, many factors influence the probability of such a result.

Q. How long does it take to build up a milk supply?

A. Opinions vary somewhat among the experts and each mother and baby will have a different experience.

Neville and Neifert suggested: "a rough estimate of the time needed to establish a full milk supply is about one week for each month preceding non nursing, plus about another week to build up an ample supply" (Neville 1983). In studies in which no galactogogues are used and there has been a lactation gap of anything from a few days to several years, the first appearance of milk has been reported within a week or so (Banapurmath et al. 1993a; Bose 1981). On the other hand, five adoptive mothers in the Indian study who received metoclopramide had not reported any milk after two weeks when they left the study (Banapurmath et al. 1993b). Where milk supply increased measurably (and sometimes it did not), it took about six weeks to get a full supply. In the studies from India and Papua-New Guinea, mentioned above—and in other non-published work in which galactogogues are used—milk production often begins and increases more quickly.

In developed countries, breastfed adopted babies often continue to have supplements until they are old enough for complementary solid foods. As they make that transition, milk supplements are usually gradually eliminated. From that point on, breastfeeding an adopted baby is scarcely different from the experience with any other baby.

Q. Why does induced lactation work so well for some women and much less well for others?

A. There is a complex mix of biological, psychological, social, and cultural factors involved in a woman's ability to produce the amount of milk her adopted baby needs. We are only beginning to understand some of these factors and to figure out how to use them to help mothers breastfeed their adopted babies. As in any other breastfeeding situation, frequent effective suckling is essential for milk production. Support within the family and from the woman's health care providers is also crucial as is the woman's belief that her body can function. As Jelliffe (1976) so elegantly put it, "Breastfeeding is a confidence game."

Chapter 8

Special Situations

Breastfeeding multiples

Breastfeeding twins (or triplets) is a unique situation. Why would anyone consider breastfeeding two or three adopted babies when adoptive breastfeeding requires so much effort? A mother who adopts more than one baby has the same reasons for breastfeeding that any other mother does. With twins or triplets, attachment and bonding take on special importance. Multiple babies are easily short-changed in the bustle of caring for them. Nurturing them at the breast is one way of ensuring that they get individual attention.

Karen Ferreira-Jorge, the South African mother whose triplets were carried to term by her mother in 1987, breastfed all three for about eight weeks. During her mother's pregnancy and for the first month after they were born, she was given tranquillizers with a galactagogue side effect. She expressed by hand and with an electric pump. As soon as the babies were born, she put them to breast every three hours although they were all rather small—her daughter weighed just under three pounds and her sons were four-and-a-half pounds, and five pounds (1.3, 2.1, and 2.3 kg) (*South Africa Sunday Times*, October 4, 1987). Her doctors prescribed a prolactin enhancer. She also used a tonic and a homeopathic tea reputed to increase milk production. Though she was disappointed not to breastfeed longer, she wrote; "I would definitely recommend it—it really brought me closer to my babies and definitely helped with the bonding even though there wasn't much milk—just the sucking helped."

Another mother, unencumbered by the publicity surrounding Karen's babies and blessed with "only" twins, managed with the help of a nursing supplementer to feed both her babies with no bottles and no solids for six months. One big help was having more than one nursing supplementer. Her husband filled an entire day's supply of plastic bags every night and set them up so they were readily available when her babies were hungry. She learned to feed them simultaneously—always a good idea when there is more than one baby—and encouraged them to suckle at the breast to fall sleep and for comfort. Eventually the babies were willing to breastfeed without the supplementer and weaned themselves—ever so slowly—around the time they were ready for preschool (Goldstein, personal communication).

In an article for *Clinical Paediatrics*, Dr. Roy Brown reported on a project in (then) South Vietnam to encourage women to become wet nurses for the

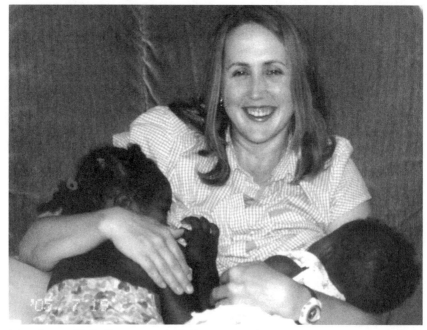

Mary Qstyn with Emily, 3 years,, and Julianna, 8 months

many orphans and abandoned infants there.

> *"Once a woman was found to be healthy and interested in providing breast milk, she would be induced to lactate. In addition to minimal cash wages she would receive three meals daily, would stay in the orphanage to assist with the care of infants, and once her milk supply was re-established would provide milk for two young orphans." (Brown 1978)*

This controlled study had to be discontinued because of the pressures during the last stages of the war there, but before it ended women were breastfeeding babies—in some cases completely feeding them with their milk. This project, like the feeding of one or more adopted babies, was not easy, but the fact that it was undertaken at all and a similar project for Bangladesh was under consideration by the World Health Organization before war there made scientific studies impractical, indicates that it is considered a feasible undertaking by many of the most prestigious segments of the medical community.

Tandem breastfeeding

Breastfeeding two babies is commonly done in tandem. One baby is born to the mother (or adopted by her) and a second one joins the family later and breastfeeds along with his older brother or sister. Jelena Brajsa, Caritas Director in Zagreb, Croatia, told the XIV International Congress on the Family about tandem nursing in its simplest form.

> *"One morning I found a box (on the doorstep) and with my leg I pushed it a little out of the way so I could open the door. But when I pushed the box I heard a cry from within—and it was a newborn baby. I was very surprised and didn't know what I should do with it, but then I remembered that a woman I knew had just had a baby, maybe fourteen days before. I went there at once . . . and suddenly she had twins!"* (Brajsa 1989)

If you are breastfeeding a very young baby when you adopt another one, a couple of weeks of feeding will probably increase your milk supply enough to meet the needs of both babies. You may even find—as one adoptive mother reported to me—that your milk supply is better with the second one than with the first. This mother breastfed her first adopted baby for eight months before her supply was adequate, adopted again while she was still feeding the first one, and had no trouble keeping pace (Hormann 1971). Her experience mirrors the experiences of some mothers who breastfeed after breast reduction surgery. Mothers who have a partial milk supply with a first baby often have more milk with any subsequent children (West 2001).

However, it doesn't always happen that way. Women who are breastfeeding older babies when they adopt a newborn may be disappointed in their hopes to fully breastfeed the new baby. The older nursling, in the process of weaning, may actually be getting relatively little milk. When a new baby is adopted, the mother might need to count on supplementing for several weeks (Auerbach and Avery 1981).

Breastfeeding without a prior pregnancy

If you have never been pregnant or never carried a baby to term you may be especially anxious to breastfeed your baby. Breastfeeding provides a substantial measure of participation in biological motherhood, and it can be very fulfilling for both mother and baby. In all probability, you will have some milk after frequent pumping or your baby's persistent suckling, but

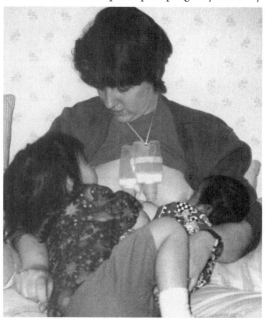

keep in mind that breastfeeding an adopted baby is not all—or even primarily—about milk.

A few mothers—usually with pituitary problems—may produce no milk at all, but these mothers have also established happy and often long-term breastfeeding relationships with their adopted babies. The babies are fed some other way—via nursing supplementer, bottle, cup, spoon, or syringe—but they are nurtured at their

Allegra and Jacob tandem nursing, each with their own nursing supplementer.

mothers' breasts. Unless you tell them, babies don't know that breasts are always supposed to supply milk; even a non-lactating breast meets their needs for sucking and closeness quite nicely. If you introduce your baby to comfort suckling at the breast, he will enjoy it as much as he would his thumb or a pacifier, probably even more because you are always there when he needs to suck or be soothed. He won't be disappointed because he won't know there is anything to be disappointed about.

Breastfeeding by another mother ("cross nursing")

Cross nursing is common in some cultures and communities, but there are risks. If another mother who is lactating well breastfeeds your baby he may be less willing to suckle at your breast when he realizes that other breasts deliver not only warmth and comfort, but food as well.

Another argument against cross nursing is its possible effect on your relationship with your baby. One major reason you are breastfeeding him is to strengthen your attachment to one another. Feeding from another mother or a series of other mothers may dilute or delay the development of that all-important bond between you.

Infection is another concern with cross nursing. Your baby is not immune to the germs another baby and his mother have—nor are they immune to his. Even a seemingly healthy baby or mother may be incubating an illness that will become apparent only after s/he has exposed other people to it. If your baby is ill, was born prematurely, or came from a developing nation, cross-infection may be of particular concern.

So, while cross nursing is—and has traditionally been—a fairly common practice, there are drawbacks. If you are considering letting someone else breastfeed your baby or putting someone else's baby to your own breast for practice, think it through carefully before you try it and satisfy yourself that there are compelling reasons to do so and that neither the mothers nor the babies involved have a communicable disease.

If you have breastfed before

If you have breastfed a baby before, you might be at some physical advantage even if you have not lactated recently because involution is never complete. Auerbach (1981) suggested that "adoptive infants were more likely

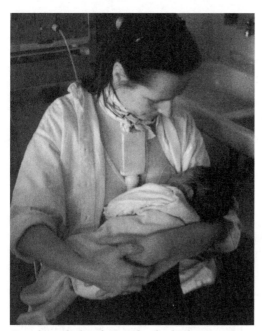

Peter breastfeeding four weeks after his heart operation, still attached to monitors and getting infusions.

to nurse if the mother had breastfed before," but did not indicate why. It may be that a woman who has breastfed before is at an advantage in understanding how lactation works and in teaching her baby to feed. She is also likely to be quite comfortable about putting her baby to breast as frequently as relactation demands.

On the other hand, the expectations of a woman who has fully breastfed in the past may be unrealistic for breastfeeding an adopted baby. She might have difficulty coming to terms with the need to supplement and she could be more vulnerable than the never-pregnant woman to being disappointed in the experience or even to feeling that she has "failed" (Riordan and Auerbach 1999; Lawrence 2005).

It is important to concentrate on the aspects of breastfeeding that are going well. Soothe your restless or fretful baby at the breast, let him fall asleep at the breast, take him into bed with you so he can feed off and on all during the night. Breastfeeding mothers do these things, casually, naturally, as a part of their relationships with their babies. While frequent feeding does have a good effect on milk supply, it is the relationship and not the milk that is the essence of adoptive breastfeeding. Even if supplements are necessary to ensure weight gain, the mother and baby who enjoy their partnership can certainly consider themselves to be breastfeeding successfully.

Breastfeeding a baby who is ill or has a disability

If your baby has health problems or has a disability, all the reasons to breastfeed apply even more strongly. In some circumstances, it may be more difficult to get the baby to take the breast. Although expectations about milk supply should be kept realistic, breastfeeding in such situations can be an important source of comfort for both mother and baby (Good 1985; Herzog and Klaus 1996; Danner 1984).

Breastfeeding a foster baby

A mother who previously breastfed her own children might want to nurture a foster baby in the same way. The child with an uncertain future should have the best possible start in life. And some very vulnerable babies in foster care may really need human milk if they are to thrive (Gribble 2005). Yet there are special factors to be considered with foster children, such as the preferences of the agency making the placement, the potential length of the foster placement, the rights of the child's biological parents, and any health concerns.

The attitudes of agencies placing babies and caseworkers can be quite variable. Some are supportive of breastfeeding. Others may consider your interest in breastfeeding a reason to deny or terminate the placement of a foster baby. Usually it is not in the baby's best interest to breastfeed if the agency objects to it—or has not been informed. If your agency doesn't support the idea, that could be very stressful for you and the baby and might defeat the whole purpose of breastfeeding—to give the baby a safe, secure start in life.

This is not to say that you cannot occasionally use the breast to soothe him, but you will not want to put him at risk for the trauma of an abrupt weaning or of undetected cow's milk allergy (if, perchance you are exclusively breastfeeding) (Hormann 1971b). Encouraging another attachment object besides your breast, such as a special blanket or a soft stuffed animal, may ease the transition away from you when he is moved.

Even agencies that are supportive of breastfeeding a foster baby will probably want you to keep the baby familiar with a bottle to facilitate the inevitable weaning. There should be adequate notice of his departure so that he can be weaned gradually (allow a couple of days at least for each feeding—more if the baby is beyond early infancy).

Sometimes, it is clear from the beginning that a foster placement is going to be a long one or it is intended that these parents adopt the child when (or if) he is released for adoption. In a long-term foster placement or one that is actually a quasi-adoption, breastfeeding can fit very well, however it may also require more than the usual amount of support.

With a short-term foster placement, you may be able to see breastfeeding as your special contribution to the baby's long-term physical and emotional health or you may decide that the effort and emotional energy needed is more than you are prepared to give for a child who will only be with you for a short time.

In some situations it may be possible to provide your foster baby with human milk from a milk bank. In the US and some European countries, human milk requires a prescription. Because some babies in foster care have special needs that respond well to human milk, you may want to explore this option with the baby's pediatrician. Your agency is unlikely to object to recommendations from the child's doctor.

In many foster placements, the preferences and rights of the biological parents must also be considered. Where reunification of the family is the goal, the agency will probably want to consult the natural parents about breastfeeding. In a pre-adoption placement, this is less likely to be the case. Do some advance research about your particular situation. You may also want to get some legal advice.

Sometimes the objection is raised that the woman who breastfeeds a foster baby is encouraging inappropriate bonding. Yet the reason children are placed in foster families rather than in group homes is to help them learn how to make attachments. Separating from foster parents and making a new attachment to adoptive parents is hard, but the child who is, by design, prevented from making attachments until the right family or circumstances come along may never be able to do it. Go ahead and love your foster baby and help him learn to love in your arms. Perhaps you will want to give him an occasional breastfeeding or decide to breastfeed him for the limited period during which you can reasonably expect to have him in your home —or perhaps not.

Talk things over with your agency first and determine together how long the baby is likely to be with you. If it looks as though he is going to leave before he would wean on his own, you will need to decide when he is going to wean—or perhaps forgo breastfeeding altogether.

Chapter 9

Support for Adoptive Breastfeeding

Your family and friends

Support is always vital to induced/adoptive breastfeeding—and support in your own household is paramount. Breastfeeding in this special situation is, for all its delights, also an added stress. Both parents really need to agree that this is what they want for their baby.

Ideally, grandparents, aunts, and uncles would be enthusiastic, too, but they might not be, just as they might not agree with some other aspect of your parenting. One of the father's tasks will be keeping critics at bay and making it clear that the parents will make the decisions about the baby's welfare and upbringing.

Having supportive friends is also helpful. If you are a single parent adopting a baby, support from at least some of your friends is essential. Prepare friends and family ahead of time so they will know what you are doing and how they can best be of help. Perhaps one or two of them could go along with you to a La Leche League or other breastfeeding support group meeting and learn with you about breastfeeding in general and adoptive breastfeeding in particular. The support of La Leche League or a breastfeeding mothers' group can be invaluable in giving you the encouragement you need, especially on days when things are not going smoothly.

Your health care providers

Having supportive health care providers for both you and your baby is so helpful it is worth making a special effort to find them. If a doctor is not actually opposed to the idea of breastfeeding an adopted baby, you can probably educate him or her enough so you will have some real help. It is common to find a doctor who has never heard of lactation being triggered by any means other than an immediately preceding pregnancy. Just a bit of documentation, a personal account, an article in a

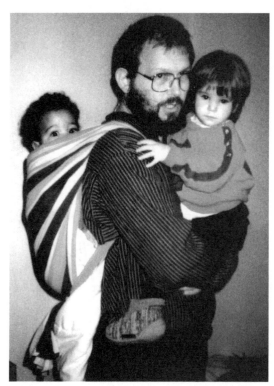

The father's support plays an important role in adoptive breastfeeding: Hannah and Peter with Rudolf Gumberger

medical journal, or a bibliography of such articles can be sufficient to spark an interest in adoptive breastfeeding. If your doctor wants to pursue it further, he or she might want to get in touch with the personal physician of another adoptive mother who has breastfed to learn more. Once they are informed, many physicians are happy to cooperate in this venture and to get some experience in an area that is unfamiliar to most medical practitioners nowadays.

Your doctor's reassurance that your baby is healthy and normal can be very important if you are worrying about whether he is getting enough to eat. It is easier to relax and enjoy breastfeeding if you aren't facing a battle with your pediatrician. And if you eventually decide against breastfeeding, you and your doctor will have the satisfaction of knowing that you had every bit of medical support you could have had.

Your adoption agency

The day may come when you will not have to consider whether or not to tell the agency that you plan to breastfeed. There are already many agencies and individual social workers interested in and supportive of adoptive breastfeeding. They frequently look for information to make available to their adopting parents—sometimes even before they have had inquiries from them. There have been some unusual instances of cooperation. One social worker arranged for the adoptive parents to be the foster parents for their baby during her agency's mandatory one-month foster care period. Lactation was already well established when their status was changed over to adoptive parents. Another social worker arranged for a baby to be dropper-fed in the hospital so he wouldn't become accustomed to a bottle before he began feeding at his adopted mother's breast.

As open adoptions become more common, adoptive parents are frequently invited to come to the birth or to the hospital shortly after the baby is born. Many adoptive mothers have begun breastfeeding within hours of their babies' birth and have been able to go home together within a day or two. This kind of interest is very encouraging. It is to be hoped that it will increase as time goes on.

Not all agencies and workers are enthusiastic about adoptive breastfeeding. With infertile couples, particularly, there is a tendency to be suspicious of motives centering on the couple's acceptance of their infertility—as if anyone could ever fully accept it. Couples have even been turned down because they have been interested in breastfeeding an adopted baby. Some have been asked to submit to psychiatric evaluation. One couple was forced to choose between a baby judged by the agency to be too old to begin breastfeeding or no baby even though they had been promised a newborn before they mentioned breastfeeding.

Because there is this unfortunate side to the picture, it is best to proceed cautiously with telling the agency. If you can get their support, that is wonderful. If not, exercise some discretion about bringing it up until breastfeeding is established and the adoption has been finalized. Certainly, the agency should be told then if the breastfeeding has been satisfying for you and your baby. You owe that much to the people who helped arrange for you to have your baby to help educate them to the possibility of this very fulfilling aspect of motherhood. Perhaps even the skeptics among them can be helped to appreciate the feelings of the adoptive mother who wrote:

> *"There are no words that can express the anguish of being told that you cannot bear children, when you have always dreamed of how you would hold your baby to your breasts—and then the joy of seeing white drops come, one at a time, and eventually become streams of milk, and the awesome wonder of nursing your adopted baby to sleep."*
> *(Hormann 1971b)*

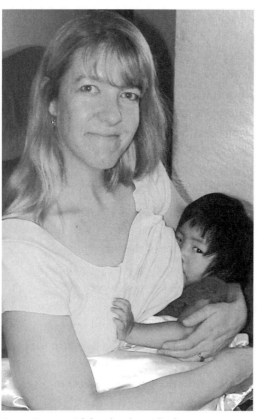

Susan Cooper with her daughter, Phoebe

Breastfeeding counseling

Adoptive mothers need specialized breastfeeding help from a counselor with experience in adoptive breastfeeding. Because there are still relatively few breastfeeding counselors or lactation consultants who have had an opportunity for experience in this area, this is frequently possible only by telephone, email, or letters.

Attending a breastfeeding support group and enlisting the support of the local group leader complements this specialized counseling and creates a day-to-day support system for the adoptive mother.

Chapter 10
What If It Doesn't Work Out?

For many reasons, you may decide breastfeeding is not a good idea for you and your baby. Perhaps the baby was quite set in his ways when he became part of your family, you got him or he doesn't really enjoy being at breast. Perhaps switching back and forth between feeding methods upsets him. You may not feel relaxed, support from your family or doctor might be lacking, or your whole situation may not be appropriate for the demands of breastfeeding an adopted baby.

Breastfeeding is a good way to grow into mothering and create a solid mother-child bond, but it is not the **only** way. Because you considered breastfeeding, even under such difficult circumstances, you are probably very aware of the needs that babies have and the signals they give to alert their parents to those needs. Everything you learned about babies when you were planning to breastfeed is just as useful to you when you bottle-feed. Your baby needs skin-to-skin and eye contact with you. He needs to be held, talked to, and touched while he is being fed. You can alternate arms so he can develop good eye-hand coordination. He can sleep in your bed and bathe with you or another family member. Using a carrier or sling to hold him close to you is just as appropriate for him as it is for a breastfed baby.

Sucking needs are important too. Keep artificial nipple holes small and throw out any that allow milk to flow out too freely. There are artificial nipples on the market that provide good exercise for the developing jaw and facial muscles. Feeding on request is best suited to most babies' needs.

The occasional pacifier can be a good thing for your baby if it isn't used to "plug him in" and keep him quiet. He might enjoy sucking on it in your arms or cradled in a carrier.

Your good mothering will help him blossom and thrive. While it is true that mother's milk is inimitable, infant formulas have improved nutritionally in recent years. They can be prepared with a minimum of fuss and bother. For the rare baby who does not thrive well on any formula, donor milk from a milk bank may be an option.

Your healthy baby probably won't need to start solids before the middle of his first year. A baby who has had a poor prenatal environment or was malnourished in the early weeks might need additions to his diet a little earlier than other babies. Artificially fed babies may have slightly different nutritional needs depending on their intake of milk products (Dewey 2005). Discuss your baby's needs with your health visitor or pediatrician, then go slowly to screen out food allergies.

Breastfeeding is ordinarily the most suitable way of feeding a baby, not just because of its nutritional uniqueness, immunological and growth factors, and practical advantages, but, just as importantly, because it is an easy natural way to provide a baby with what he needs most—tender loving care from one person, and lots of handling, rocking, and sucking. With a little foresight, your bottle-fed baby can have this kind of mothering too. Ultimately, it is the quality of mothering that provides much of the foundation for a child's development as a person.

Conclusion

Breastfeeding an adopted child is influenced by many factors and is a very special task for the adoptive family. Experiences can be quite different. If, after careful consideration of all the available information and with the support of those closest to you, you decide to breastfeed, it can be a source of great delight for you both, an experience which strengthens the mother-child bond and a time on which you and your child will later look back with very fond memories.

Appendix

The Marmet Technique of Manual Expression

The Marmet Technique of manual expression and assisting the milk ejection reflex (MER) has worked for thousands of mothers—in a way that nothing has before. Even experienced breastfeeding mothers who have been able to hand express will find that this method produces more milk. Mothers who have previously been able to express only a small amount, or none at all, get excellent results with this technique.

Technique Is Important

When watching manual expression the correct milking motion is difficult to see. In this case the hand is quicker than the eye. Consequently, many mothers have found manual expression difficult—even after watching a demonstration or reading a brief description. Milk can be expressed when using less effect methods of hand expression. However, when used on a frequent and regular basis, other methods can easily lead to damaged breast tissue, bruised breasts, and even skin burns.

The Marmet Technique of Manual Expression was developed by a mother who needed to express her milk over an extended period of time for medical reasons. She found that her milk ejection reflex did not work as well as when her baby breastfed, so she also developed a method of massage and stimulation to assist this reflex. The key to the success of this technique is the combination of the method of expression and this massage.

This technique is effective and should not cause problems. It can easily be learned by following this step by step guide. As with any manual skill, practice is important.

Advantages

There are many advantages to manual expression over mechanical methods of milking the breasts:

- Some mechanical pumps cause discomfort and are ineffective.
- Many mothers are more comfortable with manual expression because it is more natural.
- Skin-to-skin contact is more stimulating than the feel of a plastic shield, so manual expression usually allows for an easier milk ejection reflex.
- It's convenient.
- It's ecologically superior.
- It's portable. How can a mother forget her hands?
- Best of all it's free.

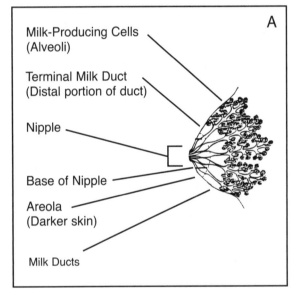

A

Milk-Producing Cells (Alveoli)

Terminal Milk Duct (Distal portion of duct)

Nipple

Base of Nipple

Areola (Darker skin)

Milk Ducts

How the Breast Works

The milk is produced in milk-producing cells (alveoli). When the milk-producing cells are stimulated, they expel milk into the duct system (milk ejection reflex).

A small portion of the milk may flow down the ducts and collect in the milk ducts under the areola known as terminal ducts (distal portion of lactiferous ducts).

Expressing the Milk

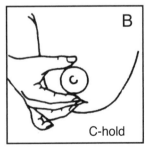

B

C-hold

Draining the Terminal Milk Ducts

1. **Position the thumb and first two fingers on the breast about 1 " to 1 1/2" (2.5 to 3.75 cm) behind the base of the nipple.**
   - Use this measurement, which is not necessarily the outer edge of the areola, as a guide. The areola varies in size from one woman to another.
   - Place the thumb pad above the nipple at the 12

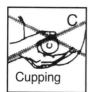
Cupping

o'clock position and the finger pads below the nipple at the 6 o'clock position forming the letter "C" with the hand, as shown. This is a resting position.
• Note that the thumb and fingers are positioned so they are in line with the nipple.
• Avoid cupping the breast.

2. Push straight into the chest wall.
• Avoid spreading the fingers apart.
• For large breasts, first lift and then push into the chest wall.

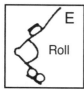
Push To Chest Wall

3. Roll thumb forward as if taking a thumbprint. Change finger pressure from middle finger to index finger as the thumb rolls forward.
• Finish Roll. The rolling motion of the thumb simulates the wave-like motion of the baby's tongue and the counter pressure of the fingers simulates the baby's palate. The milking motion imitates the baby's suck by compressing and draining the terminal milk ducts without hurting sensitive breast tissue.
• Note the moving position of the thumbnail and fingernails in illustrations D, E, and F.

Roll

4. Repeat Rhythmically to drain the terminal milk ducts.
• Position, push, roll; position, push, roll…

5. Rotate the thumb and finger position to reach other terminal milk ducts. Use both hands on each breast. Illustration G shows hand positions on the right breast.
• Note clock positions of fingers in illustration G: 12:00 and 6:00, 11:00 and 5:00, 1:00 and 7:00, 3:00 and 9:00

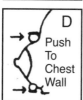
Finish Roll

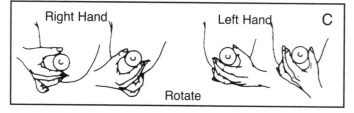
Right Hand   Left Hand   C
Rotate

Avoid These Motions
• Squeezing the breast. This can cause bruising.
• Pulling out the nipple and breast. This can cause tissue damage.
• Sliding on the breast. This can cause skin burns.

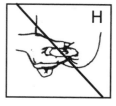
H

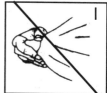
I

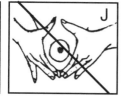
J

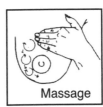

Massage

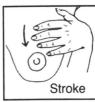

Stroke

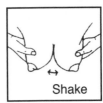

Shake

Assisting the Milk Ejection Reflex (MER)

Stimulating the flow of milk.

1. Massage the milk producing cells and ducts.
   - Start at the top of the breast. Press firmly into the chest wall. Move fingers slowly, pressing firmly in a small circular motion on one spot on the skin.
   - After a few seconds, pick fingers up and move to the next area on the breast. Do not slide on breast tissue.
   - Spiral around the breast toward the areola using this massage.
   - The pressure and motion are similar to that used in a breast examination.

2. Stroke the breast from the chest wall to the nipple with a light tickle-like stroke.
   - Continue this stroking motion from the chest wall to the nipple around the whole breast.
   - This will help with relaxation and encourage the milk ejection reflex.

3. Shake the breast gently while leaning forward so that gravity will help the milk eject.

Procedure

This procedure should be followed by mothers who are expressing in place of a full feeding and those who need to establish, increase, or maintain their milk supply when the baby cannot breastfeed.
- Express each breast until the flow of milk slows down.
- Assist the milk ejection reflex (massage, stroke, shake) on both breast. This can be done simultaneously, and only takes about a minute.
- Repeat the whole process of expressing each breast and assisting the milk ejection reflex twice more. The flow of milk usually slow down sooner the second and third time as the ducts are drained.

Timing

The entire procedure should take approximately 20 to 30 minutes when manual expression is replacing a feeding.
- Express each breast 5 to 7 minutes.
- Massage, stroke, shake for about one minute.
- Express each breast 3 to 5 minutes.
- Massage, stroke, shake for about one minute
- Express each breast 2 to 3 minutes.

Note: If the milk supply is established, use the times given only as a guide. Watch the flow of milk and change breasts when the flow gets small. If little or no milk is present yet, follow these suggested times closely. Any portion of the procedure or timing may be used or repeated as necessary.

Resources

Milk Banking Organizations

The Human Milk Banking Association of North America
1500 Sunday Drive, Suite 102
Raleigh, NC 27607 USA
919.861.4530
www.hmbana.org/
(May have information or contacts for human milk
 banks outside of North America.)

Mothers' Milk Bank
751 S. Bascom Avenue
San Jose, CA 95128 USA
408.998.4550
Fax: 408.297.9208
www.milkbanksj.org/
MothersMilkBank@hhs.co.santa-clara.ca.us

Mothers' Milk Bank at Austin
900 East 30th Street, Suite 214
Austin, TX 78705 USA
512.494.0800
877.813.MILK (toll-free)
Fax: 512.494.0880
www.mmbaustin.org/

WakeMed Mothers' Milk Bank
3000 New Bern Ave
Raleigh, NC 27610 USA
919.350.8599
Fax: 919.350.8923
www.wakemed.org/body.cfm?id=135

Mothers' Milk Bank of North Texas
1300 West Lancaster Suite 108
Fort Worth, Texas 76102 USA
817.810.0071

Mother's Milk Bank of Iowa
Department of Pediatrics, Division of Pediatric Nutrition
Children's Hospital of Iowa
200 Hawkins Drive
Iowa City, IA 52242 USA
877.891.5347
Fax: 319.353.7598
www.uihealthcare.com/depts/childrenshospitalofiowa/milkbank

BC Women's Milk Bank
C & W Lactation Services
4500 Oak Street, IU 30
Vancouver, BC V6M 3X4 Canada
604.875.2282
Fax: 604.875.2871

Mothers' Milk Bank
Presbyterian/St.Luke's Medical Center
1719 East 19th Avenue
Denver, CO 80218 USA
303.869.1888
www.health1.org/milkbank.asp

Mothers' Milk Bank
Christiana Hospital
4755 Ogletown-Stanton Road
Newark, DE 19718 USA
302.733.2340
Fax: 302.733.2602

Other resources

La Leche League International
www.llli.org/NB/NBadoptive.html
Personal stories and information about adoptive breastfeeding.

The Adoptive Breastfeeding Resource
Website only:
www.fourfriends.com/abrw/

Lact-Aid International, Inc.
PO Box 1066
Athens TN 37371-1066 USA
1.866.866.1239
1.423.744.9090
www.lact-aid.com/
Information about how the Lact-Aid nursing supplementer works, as
    well as frequently asked questions about adoptive breastfeeding and
    relactation.

Medela, Inc.
1101 Corporate Dr.
McHenry, IL 60050 USA
1.800.435.8316
1.815.363.1166
www.medela.com/
Information about the Supplemental Nursing System, as well as fre-
    quently asked questions about breastfeeding. Includes an article
    about adoptive breastfeeding written by Barbara Wilson Clay

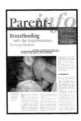

Breastfeeding with the Supplementary
Nursing System
by Marta Guoth-Gumberger, IBCLC

Additional nourishment for a baby while he is suckling at the breast
    may be the change that will make continued breastfeeding possible.
    If you want to use the SNS, this pamphlet will show you a procedure
    that is tried and tested. 16 pages with 34 colored photos. 2006.
    Available from
www.breastfeeding-support.de

References

Anderson, K. *Breastfeeding Your Adopted Baby.* LLLI, 1986.

Auerbach, K. Extraordinary breastfeeding: Relactation/induced lactation. *J Trop Pediatr* February 1981; 27:52-55.

Auerbach, K., Avery, J.L. Relactation: A study of 366 cases. *Pediatrics* 1980; 65(2):237.

Avery, J.L. in Riordan, J.A. *Practical Guide to Breastfeeding,* St. Louis: Mosby, 1983.

Avery, J. L. *Induced Lactation: a Guide for Counselling and Management,* rev ed. Athens, TN USA: Lact-Aid International, Inc., 1998.

Baker, L. What you need to know to breastfeed your baby. *Adoptive Fam* 2002; 35(6):34.

Banapurmath, C.R., Banapurmath, S.C., Kesance, N. Initiation of relactation. *Indian J Pediatr* 1993a; 30:1329-32.

Banapurmath, C.R. et al. Successful induced non-puerperal lactation in surrogate mothers, *Indian J Pediatr* 1993b; 60:639-43.

BFHI News, May/June 1999, 3.

The Bible (King James Version) Ruth 4:16.

Brajsa, J., Liebenswert sind sie alle - Leben mit verlassenen Kindern, XIV International Congress on the Family, Bonn, Germany 5 April 1989.

Black, R.F., Jarman, L., Simpson, J.B. *The Science of Breastfeeding.* Sudbury, MA: Jones & Bartlett, 1998, 227.

Brown, R.E. Relactation with reference to application in developing countries. *Clin Pediatr* 1978; 17(4):333-36.

Burgess, L.C. *The Art of Adoption.* Washington, DC: Acropolis, 1976, 8.

Da Silva, O. et al. Effect of domperidone on milk production in mothers of premature newborns: a randomized, double-blind, placebo-controlled trial. *Can Med Assoc J* 2001; 164(1):17-21.

Danner, S., Cerutti, E.R. Nursing Your Baby with a Cleft Palate or Cleft Lip, Nursing Your Neurologically Impaired Baby, Nursing Your Baby with Down Syndrome, Nursing Your Premature Baby. Rochester, New York: Childbirth Graphics, 1984.

Dewey, K. *Guiding Principles for Feeding Non-Breastfed Children 6-24 Months of Age.* WHO 2005, 20.

Duisdieker, L.B. et al. Effect of supplemental fluids on human milk production, *J Pediatr* 1985; 106:207.

The European Agency for the Evaluation of Medicinal Products (EMEA), EMEA committee for proprietary medicinal products (CPMP) Public Assessment Report. Combined oral contraceptives and venous thromboembolism. 28 September 2001. www.emea.eu.int/pdfs/human/regaffair/0220101en.pdf

FDA Talk Paper TO4-17, June 7, 2004.

Fleiss, P. Herbal remedies for the breastfeeding mother, *Mothering* 1988 48:68-71.

Gabay, M. Galactogogues: Medications that induce lactation. *J Hum Lact* 2002; 18(3):274-79.

Goldfarb, L. www.asklenore.info

Goldstein, E. Personal communication.

Gribble, K. Breastfeeding of a medically fragile foster child. *J Hum Lact* 2005; 21:42-46.

Gribble, K.D. The influence of context on the success of adoptive breast-feeding: developing countries and the west. *Breastfeeding Rev* 2004; 12(1);5-13.

Guóth-Gumberger, M. "Breastfeeding with the Supplementary Nursing System" Parent-INFO, 2006. Available from guothgum@brno.de

Guóth-Gumberger, M. Weaning from Bottle to Breast. Translated from the German. Umgewöhnung von der Flasche zur Brust. Stillnachrichten 1994 2(7), 5-14. Available from guothgum@brno.de 1992/1999

Hale, T. *Medications and Mothers' Milk*, 12th Ed. Amarillo, TX: Pharmasoft, 2006.

Hartmann, P. Control of breast function throughout the lactation cycle in women. Presented at the International Lactation Consultant Association Conference, 2002.

Herzog, C. Honigmann, K. Give Us a Little Time - How babies with a cleft lip or cleft palate can be breastfed, *Medela* 1996.

Holohan, P. "Martha" in the Irish Leader, Winter, 1983.

Hormann, E. *A Study of Induced Lactation*, La Leche League Information Sheet No. 85, 1971a.

Hormann, E. Relactation: A Guide to Breastfeeding the Adopted Baby, self-published, 1971b.

Hormann, E. and Savage, F. Relactation: Review of experience and recommendations for practice. Geneva: WHO/CHS/CAH 98.14, 1, 1998.

Hormann, E. Breastfeeding the adopted baby. *Birth Fam J* 1977; 4(4):165-73.

Humphrey, S. *Nursing Mother's Herbal*. Minneapolis: Fairview Press, 2003.

Jelliffe, D.B. Hormonal control of lactation, In Schams, D. (ed.) *Breast Feeding and the Mother*. Ciba Foundation Symposium No. 45, Amsterdam: Elsevier, 1976.

Jelliffe, D.B., Jelliffe, E.F.P. *Human Milk in the Modern World*. Oxford University Press, 1978.

Lang, S. et al. Cup Feeding: An alternative method of infant feeding, *Arch Dis Child* 1994; 71:365-69.

Lawrence, R.A. and Lawrence, R. *Breastfeeding: A Guide for the Medical Profession*. St. Louis: Mosby, 2005, 396, 727, 1117.

LLLI, Womanly Art of Breastfeeding 2004, pages 47-53.

Michaelsen, K.M. et al. Feeding and nutrition of infants and young children. Guidelines for the WHO European region, with emphasis on the former Soviet countries, WHO Regional Publications, European Series, No. 87, 140, 2000.

Minchen, M. *Breastfeeding Matters*. Alfredton, Victoria, Australia: Alma Publications, 1985, 57.

Mohrbacher, N., Stock, J. The Breastfeeding Answer Book: 3rd rev. ed. Schaumburg, IL: La Leche League International, 2003.

Morris, S. personal communication.

National Academy of Sciences, Subcommittee on Nutrition during Lactation, Committee on Nutritional Status during Pregnancy and Lactation, Food and Nutrition Board, Institute of Medicine. *Nutrition during Lactation*. Washington, DC: National Academy Press, 1991.

Nemba, K. Induced lactation: A study of 37 non-puerperal mothers. *J Trop Pediatr* 1994; 40:240-42.

Phillips, V. Non-Puerperal lactation among Australian aboriginal women (Part 1) NMAA Newsletter 1969a July-Aug; 5(4): 15-18 Reprinted as NMAA Res Bull No. 1.

Phillips, V. Non-Puerperal lactation among Australian aboriginal women (Part 2) NMAA Newsletter 1969b Nov-Dec; 5 (6): 8-9 Reprinted as NMAA Res. Bull No. 2

Prentice, A, Prentice, A. Reproduction against the odds. *New Sci* 1608, April 14, 1988.

Pryor, K. *Nursing Your Baby*. New York: Pocket Books, 1973, 111-112.

Renfrew, M., Fisher, C., Arms, S. *The New Bestfeeding: Getting Breastfeeding Right for You*. Berkeley, CA: Celestial Arts, 2000.

Riordan, J., Auerbach, K. *Breastfeeding and Human Lactation*, 2nd ed. Boston: Jones and Bartlett, 1999, 40-42, 94, 181. 557

Savage, R. Venous thromboembolism with Diane 35™ and Estelle 35™ *Prescriber Update* 2002; 23(1):2-3. www.medsafe.govt.nz/Profs/PUarticles/VTEwithCPA.htm

Schaefer, C. Personal communication.

Schaefer, C. Ed. *Drugs during Pregnancy and Lactation*. Amsterdam: Elsevier, 2001, 329.

Sunday Times (South Africa), October 4, 1987, 3.

Walker, M. *Breastfeeding Premature Babies*. Garden City Park, NY: Avery Publishing Group, 1991.

West, D. Defining Your Own Success. Schaumburg, IL: LLLI, 2001.

WHO Healthy Eating During Pregnancy and Breastfeeding: Booklet for Mothers. EUR/01 5028598 Copenhagen, 2001, 7-16.

WHO Breastfeeding counselling: A training course. WHO/CDR/93.4, 1993, 263.

Index

About La Leche League International

La Leche League International is a nonprofit organization founded in 1956 by seven women who wanted to help other mothers learn about breastfeeding. Today La Leche League is an internationally recognized authority on breastfeeding, with a mother-to-mother network that includes La Leche League Leaders and Groups in countries all over the world. A Professional Advisory Board reviews information on medical issues.

Mothers who contact LLL find answers to their questions on breastfeeding and support from other parents who are committed to being sensitive and responsive to the needs of their babies. Local LLL Groups meet monthly to discuss breastfeeding and related issues. La Leche League Leaders are also available by telephone to offer information and encouragement when women have questions about breastfeeding.

La Leche League International is the world's largest resource for breastfeeding and related information and products. The organization distributes more than three million publications each year, including the classic how-to book, THE WOMANLY ART OF BREASTFEEDING, now in its seventh edition. Look for it in bookstores, or order from La Leche League International.

LA LECHE LEAGUE INTERNATIONAL
P.O. Box 4079
Schaumburg, IL 60168-4079
847.519.7730
Fax: 847.519.0035
1-800 LA LECHE
www.llli.org

LLL Canada
Box 700
12050 Main Street West
Winchester, Ontario KOC 2KO
Canada
613.774.1842
Fax 613.774.1840
www.lalecheleaguecanada.ca

Postscript from La Leche League

La Leche League of Germany originally published this book to support the desire of adoptive mothers and mothers relactating to breastfeed their babies. We do not believe that the success of a breastfeeding relationship should be judged by the amount of milk produced, but rather by the mutual trust that develops between a mother and her child as a result of the closeness involved in breastfeeding.

What we know about relactation and induced lactation is a work in progress and you are a part of it. Our fervent wish is that you and your baby have a breastfeeding relationship that is satisfying for both of you, regardless of how you achieve that goal.

Because adoptive breastfeeding is relatively unknown in the scientific community, most of the research done on it has been in the form of case studies (observations of individual mothers) or recollections of mothers after the breastfeeding relationship has already been established. Such research tends to give less precise results than controlled studies and may be more subject to interpretation by the researchers. As a result, you may read or hear different opinions from different experts and breastfeeding counselors.

This book is primarily for adoptive parents and relactating mothers, but it was also written for all those who work with these parents and are involved in breastfeeding counseling.

La Leche League is an internationally recognized not-for-profit organization that is active in more than 63 countries with about 7000 volunteer LLL Leaders. It was founded to provide encouragement and information to mothers who want to breastfeed their babies.

An LLL Leader is specially trained by La Leche League to support mothers through regular Group meetings and through telephone counseling. She is available to parents during the entire breastfeeding period and offers both emotional support and practical help when there are difficulties. You can get in touch with an LLL Leader via the national La Leche League addresses, through the international hotline, or via the Internet at www.llli.org.

If La Leche League has been helpful to you or you would like to help us further our work, please consider becoming a member in your country or through the international organization.